The Power of the Mediterranean Diet: Lose Weight, Feel Good, and Live Longer

Table of Contents

Chapter 2:

Chapter 3:

Chapter 4:

Chapter 5:

Chapter 6:

- The Mediterranean Diet and Lifestyle

- Being active: Combining the Mediterranean diet with exercise

- Role of the Mediterranean diet in increasing energy and physical performance

- Tips for integrating the Mediterranean diet into an active lifestyle

Chapter 7:

- Meal Preparation and Recipes of the Mediterranean Diet

- Tips for meal planning and preparation

- Ideas for healthy and tasty recipes inspired by the Mediterranean diet

- Tips for shopping and ingredient selection in the Mediterranean diet

Conclusion:

- Summary of the main points covered in the book

- Encouragement to implement the Mediterranean diet for improved health and quality of life

Introduction:

Welcome to the book "The Power of the Mediterranean Diet: Lose Weight, Feel Good, and Live Longer." In these pages, we will take you on a journey to discover an ancient culinary tradition that still reveals its extraordinary potential for health and well-being today. The Mediterranean diet, with its deep roots in the culture and history of countries such as Italy, Greece, and Spain, is much more than just a dietary approach; it represents a lifestyle that promotes a balance between nutrition, pleasure, and longevity.

The Mediterranean diet stands out for its wide variety of fresh and natural foods. Based primarily on fresh fruits, vegetables, whole grains, legumes, fish, nuts, and olive oil, this diet provides the body with all the essential nutrients it needs to function at its best. At the same time, it encourages limiting the consumption of red meat, added sugars, processed foods, and saturated fats, which are associated with an increased risk of chronic diseases.

Mediterranean peoples have long understood the importance of a balanced diet not only for maintaining an ideal body weight but also for overall well-being. The Mediterranean diet is rich in antioxidants that help combat free radical damage in the body, reducing inflammation and promoting cell health. Additionally, the abundance of fiber in the diet promotes good digestion, contributing to intestinal regularity and preventing digestive disorders.

The Mediterranean diet has been extensively studied for its benefits on heart health. The high content of monounsaturated fatty acids in olive oil, combined with the presence of omega-3 fatty acids in fish, helps reduce bad cholesterol (LDL) and improve arterial health. Furthermore, moderate consumption of red wine during meals is associated with a reduced risk of heart disease due to the antioxidants present in wine.

The Mediterranean diet nourishes not only the body but also the mind. Recent studies have shown a positive correlation between a balanced Mediterranean diet and cognitive function, memory, and the prevention of neurodegenerative disorders such as

Alzheimer's. The foods rich in antioxidants, B-group vitamins, and omega-3 fatty acids in the Mediterranean diet promote brain health and keep the nervous system active.

In an era where more and more people struggle with weight-related issues and chronic diseases, the Mediterranean diet stands out as a healthy, sustainable, and flavorful dietary model. This book is designed to guide you step by step on the path to a balanced Mediterranean diet. In addition to providing a comprehensive overview of the fundamental principles of this diet, we will offer delicious tips and recipes that will make your culinary journey exciting and fulfilling. It will be an extraordinary adventure into the world of flavors, aromas, and traditions that will help you transform your relationship with food and achieve a healthy and lasting balance.

Get ready to embrace the power of the Mediterranean diet, lose weight naturally, feel pervasive well-being, and enjoy a long and vibrant life. Are you ready to embark on this extraordinary journey towards better health?

Chapter 1:

Brief Approach to the Mediterranean Diet

The Mediterranean diet is much more than a simple dietary regimen. It is a true lifestyle that embraces the balance of nutrition, pleasure, and health. To fully understand the importance and benefits of the Mediterranean diet, it is crucial to delve into its foundations, historical origins, guiding principles, key foods, and associated health benefits.

The foundations of the Mediterranean diet lie in the choice of fresh, natural, and unprocessed foods. This dietary style emphasizes an abundance of fresh fruits and vegetables, which provide essential vitamins, minerals, and antioxidants for overall well-being. The inclusion of whole grains such as whole wheat pasta, bread, and rice offers fiber and important nutrients for proper bodily function. Additionally, the Mediterranean diet emphasizes the use of healthy fats, such as olive oil, which is rich in heart-healthy monounsaturated fatty acids.

The Mediterranean diet traces its roots back to the ancient culinary traditions of Mediterranean countries, which have passed down a heritage of healthy flavors and dietary habits through generations. This diet developed within the context of a life centered around agriculture, fishing, and the gathering of local foods such as fruits, vegetables, fish, legumes, nuts, and olive oil. Mediterranean populations have enjoyed the benefits of this dietary pattern for centuries, maintaining good health and remarkable longevity.

The guiding principles of the Mediterranean diet are simple yet powerful. These principles have been identified as key components of proper nutrition within the context of the Mediterranean diet. Among these principles are the importance of a variety of fresh and seasonal foods, moderation in the amount of food consumed, attention to nutrient balance, incorporation of low-saturated-fat and low-added-sugar foods, and the habit of sharing meals with family and friends.

The key foods of the Mediterranean diet form the foundation of this healthy eating pattern. Fresh and seasonal fruits such as apples, oranges, grapes, and melons provide vitamins, minerals, and antioxidants. Vegetables like tomatoes, carrots, spinach, and bell peppers are rich in fiber, nutrients, and beneficial phytochemicals. Whole grains such as whole wheat pasta, bread, and rice provide complex carbohydrates, fiber, and nutrients. Legumes such as beans, chickpeas, and lentils are rich in plant-based proteins, fiber, and minerals. Fish, especially fatty fish like salmon, sardines, and mackerel, are an important source of heart-healthy omega-3 fatty acids. Nuts, almonds, and hazelnuts are rich in healthy fats, vitamins, and minerals. Finally, olive oil, rich in monounsaturated fatty acids and antioxidants, is the primary source of fats in the Mediterranean diet.

Numerous studies have shown that the Mediterranean diet is associated with numerous health benefits. One of the main advantages is a reduced risk of cardiovascular diseases, such as hypertension, heart attack, and stroke. This is attributed to the combination of healthy fats, antioxidants, and anti-inflammatory substances present in the Mediterranean diet. Additionally, the Mediterranean diet has been associated with a lower risk of type 2 diabetes, obesity, and certain forms of cancer, such as colon and breast cancer. The nutrients and antioxidants present in the Mediterranean diet have also been shown to promote mental health by improving mood, cognitive function, and the prevention of neurodegenerative diseases.

In conclusion, the brief approach to the Mediterranean diet provides an in-depth understanding of its foundations, historical origins, guiding principles, key foods, and associated benefits for health. This dietary style not only offers a variety of tasty flavors but can also promote overall health and long-term well-being. Implementing the Mediterranean diet can be a significant step towards a healthier and more fulfilling life.

Chapter 2:
Losing Weight, How

The Mediterranean diet not only promotes overall health but can also be a valuable ally in healthy and sustainable weight loss. In this chapter, we will explore the approach to weight loss through the Mediterranean diet, the recommended foods for promoting weight loss, strategies for portion management and calorie control, as well as examples of meal plans for weight loss.

Losing Weight with the Mediterranean Diet: The Mediterranean diet offers a balanced and sustainable approach to weight loss. It is not based on extreme restrictions or drastic diets but rather on a combination of nutritious foods and healthy habits. This approach is beneficial because it encourages the consumption of fresh, whole, and natural foods while reducing the intake of processed and high-calorie foods. The Mediterranean diet promotes a variety of foods that promote satiety, increasing the feeling of fullness and reducing the desire for excessive snacking.

Approach to Weight Loss through the Mediterranean Diet: To follow an effective approach to weight loss with the Mediterranean diet, it is important to pay attention to food choices and portion control. It is recommended to prioritize foods low in saturated fats and added sugars, such as fresh fruits and vegetables, legumes, whole grains, lean fish, and white meats. It is also important to limit the consumption of high-calorie foods such as sweets, fried foods, and sugary beverages. Additionally, adopting a balanced approach by including a combination of carbohydrates, proteins, and healthy fats in appropriate proportions is essential.

Recommended Foods for Weight Loss: The Mediterranean diet offers a wide range of recommended foods to promote weight loss. Fresh fruits and vegetables, rich in fiber and essential nutrients, can be consumed abundantly to maintain satiety while providing few calories. Whole grains, such as whole wheat bread, brown rice, and quinoa, are excellent sources of complex carbohydrates and provide sustained energy. Legumes, such as beans, chickpeas, and lentils, are rich in fiber and plant-based proteins, which contribute to satiety and stabilize blood sugar levels. Lean fish, such as cod and tuna, offer lean proteins and beneficial omega-3 fatty acids for health. Finally, low-fat dairy products, such as Greek yogurt and skim cheese, can be included in moderation to provide calcium and protein.

Strategies for Portion Management and Calorie Control: To manage portions and control calories in the Mediterranean diet, it is advisable to use some techniques. One of them is to try to eat slowly and mindfully, giving the brain time to register the feeling of satiety. It is also helpful to use smaller plates and utensils to reduce the amount of food consumed. Seasoning foods with herbs, spices, and lemon can add flavor without adding additional calories. Additionally, it is advisable to pay attention to portion sizes of fats, such as olive oil, using measuring spoons or sprays to limit the quantity.

Examples of Meal Plans for Weight Loss: Here are some examples of meal plans that can be adopted to promote weight loss with the Mediterranean diet. These are just suggestions and can be customized based on individual preferences and calorie needs:

- Breakfast: Greek yogurt with fresh fruit and low-sugar granola.

- Snack: A handful of nuts or almonds.

- Lunch: Mixed salad with grilled chicken, fresh vegetables, cannellini beans, and dressed with olive oil and lemon.

- Snack: Baby carrots with hummus.

- Dinner: Baked salmon with grilled vegetables and a portion of quinoa.

- Evening snack: Fresh fruit or a small serving of Greek yogurt.

These examples demonstrate how it is possible to create balanced and flavorful meals that promote weight loss within the context of the Mediterranean diet.

In conclusion, the Mediterranean diet offers a healthy and sustainable approach to weight loss. By using a combination of nutritious foods, strategies for portion management, and calorie control, it is possible to achieve weight loss goals without sacrificing the pleasure of eating. Implementing the Mediterranean diet as part of a healthy lifestyle can promote weight maintenance and overall well-being.

Chapter 3:

Benefits

The Mediterranean Diet not only promotes overall health but can also be a valuable ally in achieving weight loss in a healthy and sustainable way. In this chapter, we will explore the approach to weight loss through the Mediterranean Diet, the recommended foods for weight loss, strategies for portion control and calorie management, as well as some examples of meal plans for weight loss.

Feeling of Well-being with the Mediterranean Diet: The Mediterranean Diet, with its abundance of fresh and nutritious foods, promotes a sense of overall well-being. This eating pattern, rich in fruits and vegetables, whole grains, legumes, and fish, provides the body with the necessary nutrients for optimal functioning. The antioxidants present in the Mediterranean Diet help counteract oxidative stress and inflammation, promoting cell health and reducing the risk of chronic diseases. Additionally, the variety of foods and flavors characteristic of this diet stimulates the enjoyment of food and contributes to psychological well-being.

Impact of the Mediterranean Diet on Mental Health: The Mediterranean Diet has been shown to have a positive impact on mental health and mood. The high consumption of fruits and vegetables, rich in vitamins, minerals, and antioxidants, is associated with a reduced risk of depression and anxiety. The omega-3 fatty acids found in fish such as salmon and sardines are essential for brain health and may help improve mood and cognitive function. Furthermore, the Mediterranean Diet promotes good digestion and regular nutrient assimilation, which can have a positive effect on mental health and emotional balance.

Benefits for Cardiovascular Health: One of the main benefits of the Mediterranean Diet is its positive influence on cardiovascular health. The abundance of foods rich in monounsaturated fats, such as olive oil, and omega-3 fatty acids found in fish, helps reduce levels of LDL cholesterol ("bad" cholesterol) and triglycerides in the blood. Additionally, these nutrients help maintain the elasticity of the arteries, reducing the risk of hypertension and heart disease. The Mediterranean Diet, along with an active lifestyle, can contribute to maintaining optimal cardiovascular health in the long term.

Role of the Mediterranean Diet in Chronic Disease Prevention: The Mediterranean Diet is associated with a reduced risk of many chronic diseases, including obesity, type 2 diabetes, and certain types of cancer. Its richness in antioxidants, vitamins, minerals, and fiber helps protect cells from free radical damage and counteract inflammation in the body. Furthermore, the high fiber content in the Mediterranean Diet promotes good digestive health and may help prevent disorders such as constipation and intestinal diseases.

Improvement in Energy and Vitality with the Mediterranean Diet: Following a balanced Mediterranean Diet can lead to improved energy and vitality. The consumption of complex carbohydrates from whole grains, vegetables, and legumes provides sustained energy for the body. Additionally, olive oil, rich in healthy fats, can help improve cognitive function and concentration. The Mediterranean Diet also provides a range of essential nutrients, such as vitamins, minerals, and antioxidants, which are crucial for proper body functioning and maintaining high energy levels.

In conclusion, the Mediterranean Diet offers numerous benefits for overall well-being. From improving mental and cardiovascular health to preventing chronic diseases and enhancing energy and vitality, this diet represents a balanced and sustainable approach to improving quality of life. Implementing the Mediterranean Diet as part of a healthy lifestyle can lead to long-term advantages.

Chapter 4:
Fewer Risks, More Security

The Mediterranean diet not only promotes overall health but can also be a valuable ally in healthy and sustainable weight loss. In this chapter, we will explore the approach to weight loss through the Mediterranean diet, the recommended foods for weight loss, strategies for portion control and calorie management, as well as some examples of meal plans for weight loss.

Living Longer with the Mediterranean Diet: The Mediterranean diet has been associated with increased longevity and healthier aging. People who follow this diet tend to enjoy a better quality of life and have a lower incidence of chronic diseases compared to other populations. This is due to the combination of nutrient-rich foods, abundant in antioxidants, vitamins, and minerals, which promote overall health and long-term well-being.

Association between the Mediterranean Diet and Longevity: Numerous studies have shown a positive link between the Mediterranean diet and longevity. This type of diet, characterized by an abundance of fruits, vegetables, whole grains, legumes, fish, vegetable oils, and moderate amounts of red wine, provides a wide range of essential nutrients for health and vitality. The antioxidants in the Mediterranean diet help combat oxidative stress and inflammation, which are key factors in aging and the development of chronic diseases.

Impact on Cardiovascular Health: The Mediterranean diet is particularly known for its benefits on heart health and blood vessels. Regular consumption of foods such as fruits, vegetables, fish, nuts, and olive oil can help reduce the risk of cardiovascular diseases, including hypertension, atherosclerosis, and cardiac events. The omega-3 fatty acids in fish, combined with the anti-inflammatory properties of antioxidants, promote cardiovascular health by reducing inflammation, improving blood circulation, and maintaining healthy cholesterol levels.

Impact on Cognitive Health and Dementia Prevention: The Mediterranean diet has also been shown to play a significant role in promoting cognitive health and preventing dementia, such as Alzheimer's disease. The antioxidants, B-vitamins, and healthy fats present in this diet can protect the brain from oxidative stress and inflammation, maintaining optimal cognitive function. Furthermore, the Mediterranean diet promotes good blood circulation, which, in turn, contributes to better oxygen and nutrient supply to the brain, protecting nerve cells and reducing the risk of cognitive decline.

Benefits in the Prevention of Chronic Diseases: In addition to cardiovascular and cognitive benefits, the Mediterranean diet has been associated with the prevention of numerous chronic diseases. Scientific studies have highlighted that adherence to this diet can reduce the risk of type 2 diabetes, obesity, certain forms of cancer (such as breast and colon cancer), respiratory and metabolic diseases. The combination of nutrient-rich foods, antioxidants, healthy fatty acids, and fiber helps maintain metabolic balance and reduce inflammation in the body, thereby lowering the risk of developing chronic diseases.

Improvement in Energy and Vitality: The Mediterranean diet provides a balanced intake of essential nutrients, promoting increased energy and vitality. Foods rich in antioxidants, vitamins,

and minerals contribute to supporting
metabolism and providing the necessary energy
for daily activities. Additionally, the presence of
omega-3 fatty acids in fish and complex
carbohydrates in whole grains allows for a
gradual release of energy in the body, avoiding
sudden spikes and crashes. This helps maintain a
steady level of energy throughout the day,
promoting greater vitality and physical
endurance.

In conclusion, the Mediterranean diet represents a dietary approach that offers numerous benefits in reducing the risks associated with aging and ensuring greater health security. This balanced and nutrient-rich eating pattern provides the body with the necessary elements to function optimally and prevent the risk of chronic diseases. Integrating the Mediterranean diet as part of a healthy lifestyle can provide a solid foundation for a longer life, improved quality of life, and increased confidence in maintaining long-term health.

Chapter 5:

Engaging Those

Around Us

The Mediterranean Diet and Family: The Mediterranean diet is not only about individual health but can also be a valuable ally in achieving weight loss in a healthy and sustainable way. In this chapter, we will explore the approach to weight loss through the Mediterranean diet, recommended foods for promoting weight loss, strategies for portion management and calorie control, as well as examples of meal plans for weight loss.

Losing Weight with the Mediterranean Diet: The Mediterranean diet offers a balanced and sustainable approach to weight loss. It is not based on extreme restrictions or drastic diets but rather on a combination of nutritious foods and healthy habits. This approach is beneficial because it promotes the consumption of fresh, whole, and natural foods while reducing the intake of processed and high-calorie foods. The Mediterranean diet encourages a variety of foods that promote satiety, increasing the feeling of fullness and reducing the desire for excessive snacking.

Approach to Weight Loss through the Mediterranean Diet: To follow an effective approach to weight loss with the Mediterranean diet, it is important to pay attention to food choices and portion control. It is recommended to prioritize foods low in saturated fats and added sugars, such as fresh fruits and vegetables, legumes, whole grains, lean fish, and white meats. It is also important to limit the consumption of high-calorie foods, such as sweets, fried foods, and sugary drinks. Additionally, it is essential to adopt a balanced approach by including a combination of carbohydrates, proteins, and healthy fats in appropriate proportions.

Recommended Foods for Weight Loss: The Mediterranean diet offers a wide range of recommended foods to promote weight loss. Fresh fruits and vegetables, rich in fiber and essential nutrients, can be consumed abundantly to maintain satiety while providing few calories. Whole grains, such as whole wheat bread, brown rice, and quinoa, are excellent sources of complex carbohydrates and provide sustained energy. Legumes, such as beans, chickpeas, and lentils, are high in fiber and plant-based proteins, which help maintain satiety and stabilize blood sugar levels. Lean fish, such as cod and tuna, offer lean proteins and beneficial omega-3 fatty acids for health. Finally, low-fat dairy products, such as Greek yogurt and skim cheese, can be included in moderation to provide calcium and protein.

Strategies for Portion Management and Calorie Control: To manage portions and control calories on the Mediterranean diet, it is advisable to use some techniques. One of them is to try to eat slowly and mindfully, giving the brain time to register the feeling of fullness. It is also helpful to use smaller plates and utensils to reduce the amount of food consumed. Seasoning foods with herbs, spices, and lemon can add flavor without adding additional calories. Additionally, it is advisable to pay attention to the portion sizes of fats, such as olive oil, by using measuring spoons or sprays to limit their quantity.

Examples of Meal Plans for Weight Loss: Here are some examples of meal plans that can be adopted to promote weight loss with the Mediterranean diet. These are just suggestions and can be customized based on individual preferences and calorie needs:

- Breakfast: Greek yogurt with fresh fruit and low-sugar granola.

- Snack: A handful of nuts or almonds.

- Lunch: Mixed salad with grilled chicken, fresh vegetables, cannellini beans, and dressed with olive oil and lemon.

- Snack: Baby carrots with hummus.

- Dinner: Baked salmon with grilled vegetables and a serving of quinoa.

- Evening Snack: Fresh fruit or a small portion of Greek yogurt.

These examples demonstrate how it is possible to create balanced and delicious meals that promote weight loss within the context of the Mediterranean diet.

In conclusion, the Mediterranean diet offers a healthy and sustainable approach to weight loss. By using a combination of nutritious foods, strategies for portion management, and calorie control, it is possible to achieve weight loss goals without sacrificing the pleasure of eating. Implementing the Mediterranean diet as part of a healthy lifestyle can promote maintaining an ideal weight and overall well-being.

Chapter 6:
Combining Diet and Exercise

The Mediterranean Diet and Lifestyle: The Mediterranean Diet is not only a dietary pattern but also a lifestyle that promotes overall health and well-being. In this chapter, we will explore the importance of combining the Mediterranean Diet with physical exercise to achieve optimal results. We will delve into the crucial role that an active lifestyle plays in enhancing the health benefits derived from the Mediterranean diet and provide practical advice on integrating the Mediterranean Diet into an active lifestyle.

Combining the Mediterranean Diet with Exercise: Regular physical exercise is an essential component of a healthy lifestyle and can be a perfect complement to the Mediterranean Diet. Regular physical activity offers a wide range of benefits, including weight loss, improved cardiovascular health, increased energy, reduced stress, and enhanced muscle strength. When combined with the Mediterranean Diet, exercise can amplify its positive effects on health, leading to greater weight loss, improved metabolism, and better muscle toning.

Role of the Mediterranean Diet in Increasing Energy and Physical Performance: The

Mediterranean diet provides a solid foundation of nutrients that can enhance energy levels and physical performance. Foods in the diet, such as fresh fruits, vegetables, whole grains, legumes, and lean protein sources, provide complex carbohydrates, vitamins, minerals, and antioxidants that support energy, muscle efficiency, and cognitive function. Additionally, the high content of healthy fats in the Mediterranean diet, such as omega-3 fatty acids found in fish, can promote reduced inflammation, improve the body's response to exercise, and lower the risk of injuries.

Tips for Integrating the Mediterranean Diet into an Active Lifestyle: Here are some practical tips for integrating the Mediterranean Diet into an active lifestyle:

1. Exercise Planning: Schedule exercise as an integral part of your day. Find a suitable time and dedicate regular time to physical activity. Choose activities that you enjoy and that align with your fitness level, such as walking, running, swimming, practicing yoga, or participating in group classes.

2. Move More: Find opportunities to move throughout the day. Walk or bike for daily commutes, opt for stairs instead of the elevator, take active breaks during work, or organize outdoor activities with friends and family.

3. Fun Workouts: Find physical activities that are enjoyable and engaging. Explore team sports, dancing, martial arts, mountain hikes, or fitness classes that you find interesting. Variety in workouts helps maintain motivation and consistency.

4. Involve Others: Invite friends or family members to join in physical activities. Organize hikes, soccer matches, dance nights, or shared workout sessions. Group training can be a great source of motivation and fun.

5. Prioritize Recovery: Ensure you include active recovery as part of the overall approach to health and well-being. Get adequate rest, perform stretching exercises and muscle relaxation, and

dedicate time to mental recovery through activities like meditation or reading.

6. Adapt to Circumstances: Be flexible and adaptable when it comes to physical activity. Find alternatives when weather conditions or other circumstances prevent outdoor workouts. Use video tutorials or fitness apps to conveniently exercise at home.

Combining the Mediterranean Diet with regular exercise offers a holistic approach to health and well-being. Integrating an active lifestyle into the practice of the Mediterranean Diet can significantly improve outcomes in terms of weight loss, muscle toning, strength, and endurance. Furthermore, it promotes mental balance and an overall sense of well-being. Choosing activities you enjoy, being consistent, and adapting to individual needs are the keys to a sustainable and rewarding approach to combining diet and movement.

Chapter 7:

Meals and How to Approach Them

Meal Preparation and Recipes in the Mediterranean Diet: Meal preparation is a key element in successfully following the Mediterranean Diet. This chapter will delve deeper into the importance of meal preparation and provide practical tips to make this process more efficient and effective. Additionally, we will explore some healthy and tasty recipes inspired by the Mediterranean Diet, which will help you maintain variety and satisfaction in your eating habits.

Tips for Meal Planning and Preparation: Meal planning is essential for following a balanced and healthy diet. Here are some tips that will help you plan and prepare nutritious and tasty meals:

1. Weekly Planning: Set aside time each week to plan your meals. Consider the available ingredients, dietary preferences, and nutritional needs. Create a well-balanced menu that includes proteins, complex carbohydrates, healthy fats, and a variety of fruits and vegetables.

2. Grocery List: Before heading to the supermarket, create a grocery list based on your planned menu. This way, you'll be more organized and less likely to buy unhealthy or unnecessary foods. Focus on fresh and whole ingredients that are typical of the Mediterranean Diet.

3. Advance Preparation: To save time during the week, you can dedicate a day for advance meal preparation. Prepare some dishes in advance, such as soups, salads, or vegetable dishes, which can be stored in the refrigerator or frozen for consumption when you have less time to cook.

4. Portion Planning: Try to control portion sizes to avoid overeating. Use measuring tools, such as cups and kitchen scales, to assess the correct quantities of foods. Additionally, you can prepare individual servings to be consumed throughout the week, thus avoiding excessive intake.

5. Creative Cooking: Experiment with new recipes and ingredient combinations to make your meals more interesting and flavorful. Add herbs, spices, and healthy condiments to enhance the taste of dishes without adding too many calories or sodium. Make use of fresh ingredients, such as citrus fruits, herbs, and olive oil, to enrich the flavors of your dishes.

Ideas for Healthy and Tasty Recipes Inspired by the Mediterranean Diet: Here are some ideas for recipes that draw inspiration from the Mediterranean Diet:

1. Greek Quinoa Salad: Prepare a delicious salad with quinoa, tomatoes, cucumbers, red onions, black olives, feta cheese, and fresh parsley. Dress it with lemon juice and olive oil.

2. Grilled Chicken with Vegetables: Marinate chicken breast with herbs, garlic, and lemon, then grill it. Serve it with grilled vegetables, such as bell peppers, zucchini, and eggplant.

3. Tomato and Basil Pasta: Prepare a dish of whole wheat pasta and dress it with fresh diced tomatoes, garlic, basil, and a drizzle of extra virgin olive oil.

4. Baked Salmon with Potatoes and Asparagus: Bake salmon with a sprinkle of smoked paprika and serve it with baby potatoes and steamed asparagus.

Tips for Shopping and Choosing Ingredients in the Mediterranean Diet: When grocery shopping, keep in mind these tips for making healthy food choices:

1. Choose Fresh Foods: Opt for fresh fruits and vegetables, which are rich in vitamins, minerals, and antioxidants. Go for seasonal products to ensure freshness and maximum nutritional value.

2. Whole Foods: Prefer whole grains like brown rice, whole wheat pasta, whole grain bread, and

quinoa. These foods are rich in fiber and essential nutrients for your health.

3. Lean Protein Sources: Choose lean meats such as chicken, turkey, fish, and legumes to obtain high-quality protein without excess saturated fats. Include low-fat dairy products like Greek yogurt and skim cheese as well.

4. Extra Virgin Olive Oil: Use extra virgin olive oil as the primary source of fats in your cooking. It is rich in antioxidants and beneficial monounsaturated fatty acids.

Remember that meal preparation and ingredient selection in the Mediterranean Diet are fundamental to enjoying its health benefits. Harness your creativity in the kitchen to create tasty and nutritious dishes that will satisfy your palate and help you successfully follow the Mediterranean Diet.

Conclusion:

In this book, we have explored the power of the Mediterranean Diet as a comprehensive nutritional approach to achieving wellness, weight loss, and a long and healthy life. We began with a brief introduction to the Mediterranean diet, emphasizing the importance of a balanced diet for overall health and well-being.

In Chapter 1, we delved into the foundations of the Mediterranean Diet, including its historical origins and guiding principles. We discovered how this diet is based on an abundance of fresh foods, such as fruits, vegetables, whole grains, fish, legumes, and olive oil. The Mediterranean diet is rich in essential nutrients and antioxidants and is characterized by a wide variety of flavors and aromas.

In Chapter 2, we explored how the Mediterranean Diet can be a valuable tool for weight loss. This dietary approach stands out for its ability to promote a sense of satiety through the high fiber and protein content in foods.

Additionally, the Mediterranean diet encourages a reduction in the consumption of high-calorie and saturated fat-rich foods, favoring the use of healthy fats such as olive oil. We also provided practical tips for managing portions and controlling calories, along with examples of meal plans that combine the Mediterranean diet with weight loss goals.

Chapter 3 delved into the numerous benefits of the Mediterranean Diet for our overall well-being. We discovered how this eating pattern can positively influence mental health, reducing the risk of depression and anxiety. Furthermore, we highlighted the protective effect of the Mediterranean diet on cardiovascular health, helping to reduce the risk of heart disease, hypertension, and stroke. The Mediterranean diet is also associated with the prevention of chronic diseases such as type 2 diabetes and certain forms of cancer. Lastly, we emphasized how following the Mediterranean diet can lead to improved energy and overall vitality.

In Chapter 4, we explored how the Mediterranean Diet can contribute to longevity and reduce the risks associated with aging. Its combination of nutrient-rich foods and antioxidants can help prevent the accumulation of cellular damage and inflammation, factors that can contribute to premature aging and age-related chronic diseases. We also discussed the role of the Mediterranean diet in promoting good cognitive health and preventing dementia, thanks to its protective components such as omega-3 fatty acids and antioxidants.

Chapter 5 addressed the importance of involving the family in the Mediterranean Diet. We highlighted how sharing meals and adopting healthy eating habits can positively impact the health of all family members. We provided practical advice on how to involve children and adolescents in choosing healthy and tasty foods, encouraging a positive relationship with food. Furthermore, we highlighted the specific benefits of the Mediterranean diet for older adults, contributing to maintaining good health and adequate quality of life.

Chapter 6 examined the importance of combining the Mediterranean diet with an active lifestyle. We emphasized how physical exercise can enhance the benefits of the Mediterranean diet, promoting weight control, muscle toning, and cardiovascular health. We provided practical tips on how to incorporate exercise into daily routines and how to adapt nutrition to support physical activity.

Lastly, in Chapter 7, we focused on meal preparation and creating healthy and tasty recipes in the Mediterranean diet. We provided suggestions for meal planning, grocery shopping organization, and ingredient selection. Additionally, we shared ideas for recipes that showcase the fresh flavors and characteristic ingredients of the Mediterranean diet.

In conclusion, the Mediterranean Diet represents a comprehensive nutritional approach that promotes weight loss, overall well-being, and a long and healthy life. This diet is based on the habit of consuming fresh, whole, and nutritious foods, prioritizing variety and natural flavors. The Mediterranean diet promotes excellent mental and cardiovascular health, reduces the risk of chronic diseases, and enhances energy and vitality. Involving the family, adopting an active lifestyle, and preparing healthy and tasty meals are integral parts of this dietary approach. We hope that the information provided in this book has inspired readers to experience and embrace the power of the Mediterranean Diet to achieve a healthy and happy life.

Lastly, I would like to share a positive and encouraging thought. Choosing to adopt the Mediterranean Diet as a way of life is a significant step towards improving health and well-being. Remember that every person is unique and has individual needs, so it's important to consider your personal requirements and, if necessary, seek guidance from qualified professionals for specific and personalized support.

Whether you are starting your journey towards a healthier Mediterranean diet or already following this dietary pattern, I wish you the best in your path. Be patient with yourself, and remember that every small positive change counts, and each day is an opportunity to make choices that promote your health and well-being.

Continue to explore new recipes, share meals with loved ones, and enjoy the process of discovering new flavors and tastes. Maintain an active lifestyle, listening to your body and understanding its needs.

Together, we can encourage one another to follow the path towards a healthy, happy, and energetic life. Always remember that you are the main architect of your well-being, and if needed, do not hesitate to seek support from professionals experienced in the field of nutrition and health.

I wish you every success on your journey towards wellness and the joy of living. May the Mediterranean Diet be your guide to a healthy, balanced, and flavorful life.

www.ingramcontent.com/pod-product-compliance
Lightning Source LLC
Chambersburg PA
CBHW071120260726
48661CB00006B/2657